Contents

INTRODUCTION

Your pancreas helps you regulate the way that your body processes sugar. It also serves an important function in releasing enzymes and helping you digest food.

When your pancreas becomes swollen or inflamed, it cannot perform its function. This condition is called pancreatitis.

Because the pancreas is so closely tied to your digestive process, it's affected by what you choose to eat. In cases of acute pancreatitis, pancreas inflammation is often triggered by gallstones.

But in cases of chronic pancreatitis, in which flare-ups recur over time, your diet might have a lot to do with the problem. Researchers are finding out more about foods you can eat to protect and even help to heal your pancreas.

To get your pancreas healthy, focus on foods that are rich in protein, low in animal fats, and contain antioxidants. Try lean meats, beans and lentils, clear soups, and dairy alternatives (such as flax milk and almond milk). Your pancreas won't have to work as hard to process these.

Research suggests that some people with pancreatitis can tolerate up to 30 to 40% of calories from fat when it's from whole-food plant sources or medium-chain triglycerides (MCTs). Others do better with much lower fat intake, such as 50 grams or less per day.

Spinach, blueberries, cherries, and whole grains can work to protect your digestion and fight the free radicals that damage your organs.

If you're craving something sweet, reach for fruit instead of added sugars since those with pancreatitis are at high risk for diabetes.

Consider buying this book and and follow the delicious recipes for a healthy pancreas.

WHAT IS PANCREATITIS?

Pancreatitis is inflammation of the pancreas that occurs when pancreatic enzyme secretions build up and begin to digest the organ itself. It can occur as acute, painful attacks lasting a matter of days, or it may be a chronic, condition that progresses over a period of years.

TYPES OF PANCREATITIS

Acute pancreatitis refers to pancreatitis that develops suddenly, most often as a result of gallstones or alcohol ingestion. Reaction to certain medications, trauma, and infectious causes can also lead to acute pancreatitis. Acute pancreatitis can be life threatening, but most patients recover completely.

Chronic pancreatitis refers to ongoing disease in which the pancreas continues to sustain damage and lose function over time. The majority of cases of chronic pancreatitis result from ongoing alcohol abuse, but some cases are hereditary or due to diseases such as cystic fibrosis.

Approximately 87,000 people are treated for pancreatitis each year in the U.S., with the disease affecting roughly twice as many males as females. Occurring very rarely in children, pancreatitis primarily affects adults.

SYMPTOMS OF PANCREATITIS

Symptoms of acute pancreatitis include:

• Severe, steady pain in the upper-middle part of the abdomen, often radiating into the back

• Jaundice

• Low-grade fever

CAUSES OF PANCREATITIS

In more than half of patients, chronic pancreatitis is caused by long-term abuse of alcohol, which leads to damage and scarring of the pancreas. Other people may develop chronic pancreatitis as a result of hereditary causes and other causes, including:

• Gallstones

• Structural problems of the pancreatic and bile ducts

• Some medications like estrogen supplements and some diuretics

• Severe viral or bacterial infection

TREATMENT FOR PANCREATITIS

Treatment for acute pancreatitis may include nutritional support with feeding tubes or intravenous (IV) nutrition, antibiotics, and pain medications. Surgery is sometimes needed to treat complications.

OTHER TREATMENTS FOR PANCREATITIS

If your pancreas has been damaged by pancreatitis, a change in your diet will help you feel better. But it might not be enough to restore the function of the pancreas completely.

Your doctor may prescribe supplemental or synthetic pancreatic enzymes for you to take with every meal.

If you're still experiencing pain from chronic pancreatitis, consider alternative therapy such as yoga or acupuncture to supplement your doctor's prescribed pancreatitis treatment.

An endoscopic ultrasound or a surgery might be recommended as the next course of action if your pain continues.

To get your pancreas healthy, focus on foods that are rich in protein, low in animal fats, and contain antioxidants. Try lean meats, beans and lentils, clear soups, and dairy alternatives (such as flax milk and almond milk). Your pancreas won't have to work as hard to process these.

Research suggests that some people with pancreatitis can tolerate up to 30 to 40% of calories from fat when it's from whole-food plant sources or medium-chain triglycerides (MCTs). Others do better with much lower fat intake, such as 50 grams or less per day.

Spinach, blueberries, cherries, and whole grains can work to protect your digestion and fight the free radicals that damage your organs.

If you're craving something sweet, reach for fruit instead of added sugars since those with pancreatitis are at high risk for diabetes.

Consider cherry tomatoes, cucumbers and hummus, and fruit as your go-to snacks. Your pancreas will thank you.

WHAT NOT TO EAT IF YOU HAVE PANCREATITIS

Foods to limit include:

- red meat

- organ meats

- fried foods

- fries and potato chips

- mayonnaise

- margarine and butter

- full-fat dairy

- pastries and desserts with added sugars

- beverages with added sugars

If you're trying to combat pancreatitis, avoid trans-fatty acids in your diet.

Fried or heavily processed foods, like french fries and fast-food hamburgers, are some of the worst offenders. Organ meats, full-fat dairy, potato chips, and mayonnaise also top the list of foods to limit.

Cooked or deep-fried foods might trigger a flare-up of pancreatitis. You'll also want to cut back on the refined flour found in cakes, pastries, and cookies. These foods can tax the digestive system by causing your insulin levels to spike.

PANCREATITIS RECOVERY DIET

If you're recovering from acute or chronic pancreatitis, avoid drinking alcohol. If you smoke, you'll also need to quit. Focus on eating a low-fat diet that won't tax or inflame your pancreas.

You should also stay hydrated. Keep an electrolyte beverage or a bottle of water with you at all times.

If you've been hospitalized due to a pancreatitis flare-up, your doctor will probably refer you to a dietitian to help you learn how to change your eating habits permanently.

People with chronic pancreatitis often experience malnutrition due to their decreased pancreas function. Vitamins A, D, E, and K are most commonly found to be lacking as a result of pancreatitis.

DIET TIPS

Always check with your doctor or dietician before changing your eating habits when you have pancreatitis. Here are some tips they might suggest:

Eat between six and eight small meals throughout the day to help recover from pancreatitis. This is easier on your digestive system than eating two or three large meals.

Use MCTs as your primary fat since this type of fat does not require pancreatic enzymes to be digested. MCTs can be found in coconut oil and palm kernel oil and is available at most health food stores.

Avoid eating too much fiber at once, as this can slow digestion and result in less-than-ideal absorption of nutrients from food. Fiber may also make your limited amount of enzymes less effective.

Take a multivitamin supplement to ensure that you're getting the nutrition you need. You can find a great selection of multivitamins here.

ACUTE AND CHRONIC PANCREATITIS DIET COOKBOOK

DIPS

Tomato Salsa

Although salsa is most often served on chips, it's a great all-purpose condiment that can be used on burgers, sandwiches, eggs or even mixed with yogurt for a dip with a kick. Serve with endive leaves or crackers.

INGREDIENT

- 2 1/2 - 3 pounds ripe beefsteak tomatoes, seeded, if desired and finely diced 1 red onion, finely chopped

- 2 - 4 garlic cloves, minced

- 2 bell peppers, chopped (any color is fine)

- 1 jalapeno pepper or chipotle chili, seeded, if desired and finely chopped (optional) 1/3 - 1/2 cup finely chopped fresh cilantro, (about 1/2 bunch)

- 1/2 teaspoon cayenne pepper (optional) 1/2 teaspoon kosher salt

- 2 tablespoons fresh lime juice (about 1 lime)

DIRECTIONS

- Place all the ingredients in a non-reactive bowl and combine well. Cover and refrigerate at least 3 - 4 hours and up to 2 days.

Instead of the commonly used olive oil this white bean dip includes Greek yogurt. Greek yogurt has a sour taste similar to regular yogurt, but has a consistency somewhere closer to softened butter. In both the United States and Europe it has come to mean a thicker, low- moisture yogurt and can be found in the dairy section of the grocery store. Serve this dip with crudite or as a sandwich spread.

INGREDIENT

• ¼ cup assorted fresh herbs, such as parsley, basil, cilantro and/or mint leaves 2 garlic cloves

• 1 16-ounce can white beans, drained and rinsed 2 tablespoons non-fat Greek yogurt

• Juice of ½ lemon

• ¼ teaspoon kosher salt

DIRECTIONS

• Place the herbs and garlic in the bowl of a food processor fitted with a steel blade and process until well chopped. Add the remaining ingredients and process until smooth. Cover and refrigerate at least one hour and up to two days.

BREAKFAST AND EGGS

Pancakes

If you're watching your fat intake, these lower fat pancakes are perfect and if you're not, it's fine to add a bit of unsalted butter. Either way, top with real maple syrup: don't consider using the fake stuff.

INGREDIENT

- 1 1/2 cups all purpose white flour

- ¼ cup whole wheat graham flour 1/4 cup yellow cornmeal

- 1 tablespoon white sugar 1 teaspoon baking soda

- 2 teaspoons baking powder 1/2 teaspoon kosher salt

- 2 cups skim milk buttermilk 1/2 cup skim milk

- 1 large egg

• 2 large egg whites

• 1 tablespoon melted unsalted butter or canola oil

DIRECTIONS

• Place the flours, cornmeal, sugar, baking soda, baking powder and salt in a large bowl and stir to combine.

• Place the buttermilk, skim milk, egg, egg whites and butter in a small bowl and stir to combine. Add the wet ingredients to the dry ingredients and mix until just combined. Do not over- mix.

• Place a large non- stick skillet over a medium heat and when it is hot, drop ladlefuls of batter on the surface. Cook until bubbles form. Flip over and cook for about 2 minutes. Serve immediately with real maple syrup.

Steel Cut Oats with Cranberries and Walnuts

There is no question that steel cut oats are far better – in flavor, texture and taste- than rolled oats. However, the common complaint- that they take forever to cook- is a fair one. My solution: start the process the night before!

This recipe serves one but can easily be quadrupled.

iNGREDIENTS

• 1/3 cup steel cut oats 1 1/3 cup water

• To each serving add:

• 2 tablespoons skim milk

• 1 tablespoon dried cranberries, raisins, dates, apricots or cherries

• 1 teaspoon lightly toasted chopped walnuts, pecans or almonds (optional) 1 teaspoon ground flax seed (optional)

• ½ teaspoon wheat bran

• 1 teaspoon maple syrup, brown sugar or honey Other options, per serving:

• apples and cinnamon sugar blueberries

DIRECTIONS

• The night before: Place the oatmeal and water in a small saucepan and bring to a boil over high heat. Cover and cool to room temperature. Refrigerate overnight.

• The next morning: Remove the cover, place the saucepan over high heat and bring to a boil. Reduce the heat to low, partially cover and cook until the oatmeal is tender, 10- 15 minutes. Add the milk, cranberries, nuts, flax, wheat and maple syrup, as desired. Serve immediately.

Apple Banana Smoothie

Smoothies are infinitely adaptable but here is my basic and most favored version. Feel free to substitute peaches or pears for the apple, and apple or pineapple juice for the orange. I always use bananas; they are indispensable for the smooth texture and creamy mouth-feel they impart. Add nuts or ground flax seed if your diet allows.

INGREDIENT

• 1 over-ripe banana, cut in 4

- 1 Granny Smith apple, cored and chopped 1 cup non-fat plain yogurt

- 1/2 cup orange juice

- ½ cup water

- 1 tablespoon wheat germ or wheat bran 1 tablespoon ground flax seed (optional)

DIRECTIONS

- Place the banana and apple in a blender or the bowl of a food processor fitted with a steel blade and process until almost smooth. Add the remaining ingredients and process until smooth. Serve immediately or refrigerate up to one hour.

French Toast

Almost entirely fat free, this version of French Toast can be adapted to almost any kind of bread. Experiment with whatever kind you like best: just be sure it is day old, so that it absorbs the liquid but can still keep its shape. Serve with real maple syrup, your favorite jam or jelly, apple sauce or stewed fruit, or sprinkled with cinnamon –sugar.

INGREDIENT

• 3/4 cup skim milk

• 2 large egg whites 1 large egg

• 1/4 teaspoon vanilla extract 1/8 teaspoon
ground cinnamon

• 6 slices oatmeal or cinnamon raisin bread, day
old

DIRECTIONS

• Place the skim milk, egg whites, egg, vanilla
extract and cinnamon in a large mixing bowl and
stir until just combined.

• Place a large non- stick skillet over medium
heat and when it is hot, dip the bread, on slice at
a time in the egg mixture. Place the bread on the
skillet and cook until golden brown on both sides,
about 3 minutes. Repeat with all the bread. Serve
immediately with real maple syrup.

Spinach and Cheese Frittata

The frittata, an open-faced omelet, is one of my
favorite dishes: easy to make, infinitely

adaptable, full of protein and great for breakfast, brunch, lunch and even a light dinner.

INGREDIENT

• 1 teaspoon vegetable or olive oil 1 large Spanish onion, chopped 2 garlic cloves, minced

• 6 large eggs, lightly beaten

• 10 large egg whites, lightly beaten

• 2 cups tightly packed flat leaf spinach, chopped or baby spinach, well washed 1/2 cup crumbled non-fat feta cheese or goat cheese

• 1 teaspoon kosher salt

• ½ teaspoon black pepper

DIRECTIONS

• Place a non stick skillet over medium heat and when it is hot, add the oil. Add the onion and garlic and cook, stirring occasionally, until they are fragrant, soft and slightly caramelized, about 8- 12 minutes (depending on the size of the pan). Set aside to cool.

• Add the remaining ingredients and mix well. The mixture will look very spinach-y and not very egg-y. (The frittata can be completed up to this point the night before. Simply cover and refrigerate).

• Preheat the oven to 350 degrees. Place a lightly buttered non stick 9 inch square pan in the oven and when both are hot, add the egg mixture and let cook until the eggs are set, 15- 20 minutes.

• Serve hot, room temp or cold with a little bit of fruit salad on the side or Mesclun greens.

Granola

Granola is a great food for snacking, to eat as cereal or as an add-in to yogurt or cottage cheese. Commercial versions are often high in fat and very expensive; why not make your own personalized version for far less?

INGREDIENTS

• 2 cups old fashioned oats

• ½ cup wheat germ

• ½ cup wheat bran

• 1/4 cup pecans or walnuts, coarsely chopped 1/4 cup almonds, chopped or sliced

• ¼ cup flax seed

• ½ teaspoon kosher salt

• 6 tablespoons maple syrup or honey 1/3 cup egg whites

• 2 tablespoons canola oil 1 teaspoon vanilla extract

• ½ cup raisins

• ½ cup dried cranberries

• ½ cup chopped dried apricots

DIRECTIONS

• Preheat the oven to 275 degrees. Line a baking sheet with parchment paper.

• Place the oats, wheat germ, wheat bran, nuts, flax seed and salt in a medium size bowl and mix to combine. Add the maple syrup, egg whites, oil and vanilla and mix again. Pour onto the prepared baking sheet. Pat down to form an even layer, making sure the mixture is neither too thick nor too thin. Transfer to the oven and cook for 15 minutes. Remove the pan from the oven and flip over, in chunks. Return to the oven and bake for 15 minutes. Turn off the oven and let the pan stay in the oven for 30 minutes. This will help the mixture dry out but not overcook. Add the dried fruit, mix well and set aside to cool. Transfer to an air-tight storage container.

Baked Broccoli Frittata

Frittatas are a perfect meal. Good for kids and adults, they can be whipped up in minutes and served hot, cold or at room temperature. They can be filled with just about anything: herbs, vegetables, meats and/or cheeses.

INGREDIENTS

- 2 teaspoons olive or canola oil

- 1 small Spanish or purple onion, coarsely chopped 2 garlic cloves, finely chopped

- 3 cups chopped broccoli florets or zucchini 4 large eggs, lightly beaten

- 4 large egg whites, lightly beaten 1 cup grated cheese (optional)

- 1 cup non- fat sour cream, yogurt or ricotta cheese

- 2 cups cubed day old bread, diced and cooked potatoes or leftover pasta 2 teaspoons kosher salt

DIRECTIONS

- Preheat the oven to 350 degrees. Lightly grease an 8 inch springform pan or 10 inch pie plate.

- Place a small pan over a medium low flame and when it is hot, add the oil. Add the onion and garlic and cook until the onion is translucent, about 10 minutes. Add the broccoli and cook until soft, about 10 minutes. Set aside to cool slightly.

- Place the remaining ingredients in a mixing bowl and mix, by hand; add the cooled broccoli mixture. The frittata can be completed up to this point the night before. Simply cover and refrigerate.

- Preheat the oven to 350 degrees.

- Place a lightly buttered non stick 9 inch square pan in the oven and when both are hot, add the egg mixture and let cook until the eggs are set, 15- 20 minutes.

• Serve as it is or with salsa

SALADS

Farro Panzanelle

Inspired by Italian bread salads, this salad substitutes bread with farro, a delicious, slightly chewy whole grain. If you can't find it, spelt or soft wheat berries are similar and equally delicious.

INGREDIENTS

• ½ cup farro 2

• 2 large or 3 beefsteak tomatoes (about 2 ½ cups diced)

• ¾ cup diced English cucumber

• ¼- 1/3 cup diced red onion (about ¼ medium)

• ¼ cup scallions, thinly sliced

• 2 tablespoons chopped fresh basil leaves

• 1/2 cup chopped fresh Italian flat leaf parsley leaves 1 tablespoon extra-virgin olive oil

• 1 ½ teaspoons red wine vinegar Kosher salt and black pepper to taste

DIRECTIONS

• Fill a small saucepan with water and bring to a boil over high heat. Add the farro and cook until it is tender, 15- 20 minutes. Drain. Transfer to a large mixing bowl and set aside to cool to room temperature.

• Add the tomatoes, farro, cucumbers, onion, scallions, basil and parsley and gently mix. Add the oil, vinegar, salt and pepper and gently mix again.

Tuscan Bread Salad

This brilliant and classic Italian dish, minus the olive oil, should be made in the summer when tomatoes are at their peak!

INGREDIENTS

• 2 cups day old French or sourdough bread, cubed 2 medium Beefsteak tomatoes, diced

- 1 English cucumber, halved and thinly sliced 1/4 cup coarsely chopped fresh chives

- 1 bell pepper, any color, cubed

- 1/4 cup coarsely chopped fresh basil leaves 1 tablespoon finely chopped fresh oregano

- 1/2 cup coarsely chopped fresh Italian flat leaf parsley leaves 1 - 2 garlic cloves, finely chopped or pressed

- 1 - 2 tablespoons red wine vinegar 1/2 teaspoon kosher salt

- 1/4 teaspoon black pepper 1 - 2 tablespoons olive oil

DIRECTIONS

- Place bread, tomatoes, cucumber, chives, bell pepper, basil, oregano and parsley in a large non-reactive mixing bowl.

- Place garlic, vinegar, salt, pepper and oil in a bowl and mix well. Drizzle over vegetables. Cover and refrigerate at least 4 hours.

A more elaborate take on the classic Greek Salad. With some whole wheat pita and White Bean Dip (page 00), this is a tasty lunch or hot weather dinner.

INGREDIENTS

• 1 head romaine lettuce, pale green inner leaves only 3 cups baby spinach leaves

• 1 Beefsteak tomato, cubed

• ½ English cucumber, cubed

• 1 small red onion, thinly sliced

• ¼ cup raisins or dried figs, chopped 1

• ½ tablespoons fresh lemon juice 1 ½ tablespoons olive oil

• 1 teaspoon dried Greek oregano

• ½ teaspoon kosher salt

• ¼ teaspoon black pepper

• 1/3- ½ cup crumbled non-fat feta cheese

DIRECTIONS

• Place the romaine, spinach, tomato, cucumber, red onion, and raisins in a large salad bowl and toss to combine.

• Place the oil, vinegar, oregano, salt and pepper in a small bowl and whisk together. Pour over the salad, gently toss, sprinkle with the feta cheese and serve immediately.

Curried Tuna

Instead of bread, try wrapping a scoop of tuna in a romaine leaf. Consider substituting the apple with an orange, peach or mango and the currants with dried apricots, dates or cranberries.

INGREDIENTS

• 9 ounces white tuna in water, drained well 1 tablespoon non-fat or low fat yogurt

• 1 tablespoon non-fat or low fat sour cream 1 tablespoon non-fat to low-fat mayonnaise 2 tablespoons Major Grey's mango chutney 1 teaspoon curry powder

• 1/2 Granny Smith apple, peeled, if desired, cut in small dice 1/4 cup currants or raisins

DIRECTIONS

• Place all the ingredients in a mixing bowl and stir until just combined. Cover and refrigerate at least one hour and up to overnight.

Buttermilk Dressing
A great all- purpose dressing for greens. Yield: about ½ cup (info per 1 Tablespoon=) 1 garlic clove

INGREDIENTS

• 1/4 cup non-fat buttermilk

• 2 tablespoons red wine vinegar 1 tablespoon olive oil

• 1 tablespoon freshly chopped mint, dill or tarragon (optional) Kosher salt and black pepper to taste

DIRECTIONS

• Place the garlic, buttermilk and vinegar in a blender or a food processor fitted with a steel blade and process. While the machine is running, gradually add the oil. If desired, add herbs by hand. Add salt and pepper to taste. Use immediately or cover and refrigerate up to two days.

Five Bean Salad with Mustard Vinaigrette

This tangy, yet buttery salad makes a great lunch dish: simply serve it on chopped romaine or mesclun.

INGREDIENTS

• 1/2 cup each red kidney, black, white beans, garbanzo or fava beans (2 cups beans in total, any combination is fine)

• 2 cups green beans, trimmed and snapped in half

• 1/2 bunch scallions, root end and 1 inch of green part trimmed and discarded, remainder chopped

• ¼ cup coarsely chopped Italian flat leaf parsley

• 2 garlic cloves, finely chopped 2 tablespoons red wine vinegar 2 tablespoons Dijon mustard

• 2 tablespoons olive oil

• 4 tablespoons chopped fresh basil leaves

DIRECTIONS

• Place the beans, scallions and parsley in a medium size mixing bowl and toss to combine. Set aside.

• Place the garlic in a food processor or blender and pulse until the garlic is chopped. Add vinegar, mustard and basil and mix until well combined. With the machine running, slowly add oil. Add salt and pepper to taste. Pour the dressing over the beans and refrigerate for at least two hours to let the flavors meld. Serve cold or at room temperature.

White Bean and Tuna Salad

A take off on the classic Italian salad, this protein packed version is lighter but equally flavorful. Consider serving on a bed of arugula or watercress.

For the dressing:

• ¼ cup fresh lemon juice

• ¼ cup olive oil

• ½ teaspoon black pepper 1 teaspoon Dijon mustard

For the salad:

• 2 cans (6 ½ ounces each) white tuna in water, drained well 2 cups cooked or canned cannellini beans, rinsed well

• ½ small red onion, thinly sliced

• ½ cup chopped Italian flat leaf parsley leaves 1 cup diced English cucumber

DIRECTIONS

• To make the dressing: Place the lemon juice, olive oil, pepper and mustard in a bowl and using a whisk, combine well. Set aside.

• Place the tuna, beans, onion, parsley and cucumber in a large bowl and gently toss. Add the dressing and toss again. Transfer to a container, cover and refrigerate at least 1 hour and up to overnight.

This classic French vegetable combo makes a great side dish, hot or cold, a topping for burgers, a filling for omelets or crepes, a vegetarian main dish—the use is only limited by your imagination.

INGREDIENTS

• 1 tablespoon olive oil

• 1 Spanish or red onion, chopped 4 garlic cloves, minced

• 1 medium eggplant, peeled and diced 4 small or 2 large zucchini, diced

• 1 red bell pepper, diced

• 2 cups diced tomatoes, canned or fresh 1 lemon, quartered

• 1 tablespoon parmesan cheese

• 2 tablespoons chopped fresh basil leaves

DIRECTIONS

• Place a medium size stockpot over medium low heat and when it is hot, add the oil. Add the onion and garlic and cook 10 minutes. Add the eggplant and zucchini, cover and cook 10 minutes. Add the red pepper and cook, covered, for 10 minutes. Add the tomatoes and cook, uncovered, for 10 minutes, if they are canned and 20 minutes, if fresh.

• Cover and refrigerate overnight or serve immediately, garnished with lemon quarters, Parmesan cheese and basil.

SOUPS

Tropical Gazpacho

A slight variation from traditional gazpacho makes this tropical version a little unusual and very special. Gazpacho makes a great first course for a light dinner, the main course for lunch or alone for a midday snack.

INGREDIENTS

• 6 plum tomatoes, cut in small dice

• 2 red, orange or yellow bell peppers, cut in small dice 1 English cucumber, cut in small dice

• 2 thick slices fresh pineapple, peeled and cut in small dice (about 1 1/2 cups) 1 fresh mango, peeled, pitted and cut in small dice

- 1/4 cup finely chopped fresh basil leaves 1/2 red onion, minced

- 1/4 cup red wine vinegar 2 cups V8 or tomato juice

DIRECTIONS

- Place all the ingredients in a large non-reactive bowl and mix well. Cover and refrigerate at least two hours and up to overnight.

Minestrone

This recipe makes a large amount of minestrone because if you're going to spend all the time, you might as well get several meals out of it. We suggest freezing portion sizes for a quick lunch or light dinner.

INGREDIENTS

- 1 tablespoon olive oil 1 Spanish onion,

- chopped 2 garlic cloves, minced

- 3 carrots, chopped

- 1 celery stalk, chopped

- ½ fennel bulb, chopped

- ¼ teaspoon dried fennel

- ¼ teaspoon dried rosemary 1 bay leaf

- 10 cups non-fat chicken stock 1 ham hock (optional)

- 1 16 ounce can diced tomatoes, drained 2 ½ cups cooked or canned white beans 1 zucchini, diced

- 1 ¼ cup (3 oz) green beans, trimmed and halved

- ½ bunch kale, leaves coarsely chopped

DIRECTIONS

- Place a large stockpot over medium heat and when it is hot, add the oil. Add the onion, garlic, carrots, celery and chopped fennel and cook, stirring occasionally, until all have softened but not browned, 15- 20 minutes. Add the dried fennel, rosemary and bay leaf and cook 5 minutes. Add the chicken stock, ham hock and diced tomatoes and bring to a gentle boil. Lower the heat to low and cook until the broth is no longer clear and all the ingredients have come together, about 2 hours. Add the white beans, zucchini, green beans and kale and cook until softened but not mushy, 20- 30 minutes. Set aside to cool for 20 minutes. Transfer to a container, cover and refrigerate overnight. Remove the bay leaf before serving.

Mushroom Barley Soup

The combination of mushrooms and barley give this soup a rich, almost meaty flavor and texture. Add some bread and you have your dinner!

INGREDIENTS

• 1 Spanish onion, chopped 3 garlic cloves, chopped

• 2 carrots, chopped

• 1 celery rib, chopped

• 1 pound button mushrooms, halved and sliced

• ½ teaspoon dried thyme

• 10 cups non-fat chicken broth 1/2 cup barley

• ½ teaspoon balsamic vinegar or fresh lemon juice 1 tablespoon fresh thyme leaves

DIRECTIONS

• Place the onion, garlic, carrot, celery, mushrooms, thyme and 1 cup chicken broth in a large stockpot and cook, stirring occasionally, until all have softened, 15- 20 minutes. Add the remaining chicken broth and barley and bring to a gentle boil. Lower the heat to low and cook until the barley has softened and the soup starts to come together, about 2 hours. Set aside to cool for 20 minutes, add the balsamic vinegar and thyme and stir well. Transfer to a container, cover and refrigerate overnight.

Roasted Butternut Squash with Apples

Rich, luscious and creamy and yet no cream and very little fat. A great

INGREDIENTS

• 1 large butternut squash, peeled, seeded and cubed 1 Granny Smith apple, peeled, if desired, and cubed 1 tablespoon water

• 1 Spanish onion, chopped 2 garlic cloves, chopped

• 2 teaspoons curry powder 1 teaspoon dried basil

• 8- 9 cups non-fat chicken or vegetable stock Preheat the oven to 425 degrees.

DIRECTIONS

• Place the squash and apple cubes on a sheet pan and sprinkle lightly with water. Transfer to the oven and bake until the squash is browned and tender, about 40 minutes.

• When the squash is almost done, place a stockpot over medium heat and add the water, onion, garlic, curry and dried basil and cook until the onion is tender, about 5- 7 minutes.

• Add the roasted squash and apples and the stock and bring to a boil. Lower the heat to medium low and cook for 20 minutes.

• Transfer to a blender, in batches and blend until smooth. Transfer to a container, cover and refrigerate up to 3 days or serve immediately.

Simpler and quicker than using a whole chicken, this homey bright chicken soup is worthy of Grandma.

INGREDIENTS

• 1 small onion, coarsely chopped

• 3 carrots, halved lengthwise and thinly sliced 2 celery stalks, halved lengthwise and sliced 10 cups non-fat chicken stock

• 1 bay leaf

• one strip lemon zest

• 2 medium potatoes, cut in small dice (about 2 cups) 2 cups shredded or diced cooked skinless chicken

• 1 tablespoon fresh thyme leaves

DIRECTIONS

• Place the onion, carrots, celery and ¼ cup stock in a large stockpot over medium heat and cook until the vegetables are tender, about 10- 15 minutes. Add the remaining stock, bay leaf and lemon zest and cook over low heat for 1 hour.

• Place the potatoes in a separate pot, cover with cold water and bring to a boil over high heat. Cook until the potatoes are tender, about 20 minutes. Drain and reserve.

• Add the potatoes, cooked chicken and thyme to the soup and serve immediately or cover and refrigerate for up to 2 days.

Vegetable Chili

Lighter than the classic beef chili, this rendition is rich in vegetables and heart healthy beans. Feel free to vary the beans as you like.

INGREDIENTS

• ½ cup water

• 2 Spanish onions, coarsely chopped 4 garlic cloves, finely chopped

• 2 bell peppers, any combinations of colors, seeded and coarsely chopped 1 small eggplant, peeled, if desired, and cubed or 3 zucchini, cubed

• 1 tablespoon dried Greek oregano 1 - 2 tablespoons chili powder

- 2 teaspoons crushed red pepper flakes

- 1 tablespoon ground cumin, or more, to taste

- 1 teaspoon cayenne pepper (optional)

- 1 16 ounce can or 2 cups cooked white beans, rinsed and drained 1 16 ounce can or 2 cups cooked black beans, rinsed and drained 4 (1 pound) cans dark red kidney beans, rinsed and drained

- 1 cup dried lentils, washed and picked over for stones

- 2 20 ounce cans whole tomatoes, coarsely chopped, including juice Freshly chopped cilantro or basil

DIRECTIONS

- Place the water, onions, garlic, peppers, eggplant or zucchini and spices in an 8 quart stockpot over low heat and cook until the vegetables are softened, 10- 15 minutes.

- Lower the heat to low, add the beans, lentils and tomatoes and cook, covered, for 1 - 2 hours, stirring occasionally. Cover and refrigerate at least overnight and up to five days. Or freeze in serving sizes up to two months.

• Just prior to serving, add basil or cilantro.

Lauren's Cauliflower Soup

Soup doesn't get simpler than this embarrassingly easy, non- fat soup. Food doesn't get plainer than this so feel free to add curry powder, a tiny bit of cream or Parmesan cheese if your diet allows, fresh basil or cilantro leaves or some Dijon mustard.

INGREDIENTS

• 1 Spanish onion, chopped

• 5- 6 cups non-fat chicken stock

• 1 head cauliflower, cored and chopped

DIRECTIONS

• Place the onion and 2 tablespoons stock in a large saucepan over medium heat and cook until the onion gets very tender and starts to brown, about 10 minutes. Add the remaining chicken stock and bring to a boil. Lower the heat to low, cover and cook until the cauliflower is tender, about 35 minutes. Remove the solids and transfer to a food processor or blender.

• Process, in batches, until smooth, gradually adding the remaining broth. Transfer to a container, cover and refrigerate up to 2 days or serve immediately.

Carrot Soup with Ginger

Simple and inexpensive to make, silky, rich and filling, served hot or chilled, Carrot Soup with Ginger makes a great lunch, afternoon pick-me-up, or when accompanied by salad, a light dinner.

INGREDIENTS

• 1 tablespoon water

• 1 medium Spanish onion, coarsely chopped 1 pinch ground cinnamon

• 2 teaspoons fresh ginger root, peeled and coarsely chopped 2 pounds carrots, sliced

• 1 Granny Smith apple, peeled, if desired and diced 8 cups non-fat chicken stock

• 1/2 cup non- fat buttermilk or yogurt (optional)

DIRECTIONS

• Place the water, onion, cinnamon, ginger root, carrots and apple in a heavy bottomed saucepan or stockpot over medium low heat and cook until the they are beginning to soften, about 15- 20 minutes.

• Add the chicken stock, raise the heat to high and bring the soup to a boil. Reduce the heat to low and cook for 30 minutes.

• Transfer the soup to a blender and process until completely smooth, gradually adding the buttermilk, if desired. Serve immediately or cover and refrigerate up to 5 days.

Lentil Barley Soup

Make this your standard lentil soup but vary the vegetables by substituting leeks or shallots for the scallions, adding zucchini or kale and replacing the barley and quinoa with brown rice for a slightly nutty flavor.

INGREDIENTS

• 1 cup dried lentils, rinsed and picked over 4 scallions, including greens, sliced

• 5 carrots, chopped

• 3 celery stalks, including leaves, chopped 1 teaspoon dried Greek oregano

• 1/4 cup barley

• 1/4 cup quinoa, rinsed

• 10- 12 cups non-fat chicken or vegetable stock

• 1 16 ounce can diced tomatoes, including liquid Kosher salt and black pepper to taste

• 1 tablespoon red wine vinegar or lemon juice

DIRECTIONS

• Place the lentils, scallions, carrots, celery stalks, oregano, barley, quinoa and chicken stock in a 6 quart pot and bring to a boil over a medium high heat. Reduce the heat to low and simmer, uncovered, for two hours.

• Add the tomatoes and continue cooking for an additional one to two hours. Add salt and pepper to taste. Just prior to serving, add vinegar.

RICE, POTATOES AND GRAINS

Beans and Rice

Favored for its meatless high protein count, this traditional combination can be found in many different ethnic cuisines. Feel free to increase the spices, if your diet allows it.

- INGREDIENTS

- 2 teaspoons olive oil

- 2 garlic cloves, pressed or finely chopped 1 small onion, chopped

- 1 red bell pepper, seeded and diced

- 1/4 teaspoon cayenne pepper, or more to taste 1/8 teaspoon cumin, or more to taste

- 1 fresh or canned tomato, coarsely chopped

- 1 16 ounce can black beans or red kidney beans, drained and rinsed 1 - 2 cups water, non-fat chicken or vegetable stock

- 3 - 4 cups cooked white or brown rice Salt to taste

• 2 tablespoons freshly chopped cilantro (optional) or chopped Italian flat leaf parsley leaves

DIRECTIONS

• Place a large skillet over medium low heat and when it is hot, add the oil. Add the garlic, onion, bell pepper, cayenne and cumin and cook until the onion has softened, about 10 minutes. Reduce the heat to low, add the tomato, beans and water and cook until the beans are very soft, about 20 minutes. Add salt to taste. Serve immediately over rice and garnished with the cilantro if desired.

Overstuffed Broccoli Parmesan Potatoes

For a quick meal, roast the potatoes ahead of time and assemble just prior to eating. Feel free to substitute kale, escarole, cauliflower or broccoli rabe for the broccoli.

INGREDIENTS

• 4 Idaho potatoes, pricked with a fork 1 cup non fat Greek yogurt

• 1/2 cup grated Parmesan cheese

• 2 scallions, trimmed, white and green thinly sliced 1/2 teaspoon kosher salt

• 1/4 teaspoon dry mustard pinch cayenne

• ¼ head broccoli, lightly steamed, florets chopped, stalks peeled and finely chopped Hungarian paprika

DIRECTIONS

• Preheat the oven to 400 degrees.

• Place the potatoes in the oven and roast until the flesh is tender and the skin is slightly hardened, about 40 minutes. Set aside for 10 minutes.

• Lay the potatoes on a cutting board and cut off the uppermost ¼. Discard the top. Scoop out the flesh and place it in a medium size mixing bowl. Add the yogurt, parmesan cheese, scallions, salt, mustard and cayenne and mix until well combined. Add the broccoli and mix again. Divide into 4 portions and return the mixture to the scooped out potatoes. Sprinkle with paprika, transfer to the oven and bake until heated throughout, about 15 minutes. Serve immediately.

Roasted Mixed Vegetables

Oven roasting is a simple, no fuss way to intensify the flavor of vegetables. It t is a method that works well for just about every variety.

INGREDIENTS

• 1 large red onion, sliced or 4 shallots1 1 red bell pepper, seeded and sliced 1 yellow squash, sliced

• 1 zucchini, sliced diagonally 2 cups cherry tomatoes

• 4 - 8 garlic cloves, in paper

• 1 teaspoon dried thyme, basil or rosemary 1/4 - 1/2 teaspoon kosher salt

• 1/4 teaspoon black pepper 1 tablespoon olive oil

• 1 tablespoon balsamic vinegar

DIRECTIONS

• Preheat the oven to 400 degrees. Line the pan with parchment paper or a silpat.

• Put all the ingredients, except for the balsamic vinegar, in a baking pan and toss well. Transfer to the oven and roast until the vegetables are browned and tender, about 1 hour. Do not crowd the pan: if necessary use two!

• Transfer the vegetables to a shallow bowl and sprinkle with balsamic vinegar. Serve immediately.

Roasted Beets with Orange and Fresh Mint

Even beet detractors will love this side dish. Roasting the beets enhances their natural sweetness and richness. Don't like mint? Simply omit it or substitute basil.

INGREDIENTS

• 2 bunches beets, trimmed, greens discarded or saved for another use 2 teaspoons olive oil

• 3 tablespoons orange juice 4 tablespoons balsamic vinegar 1 teaspoon Dijon mustard

• 2 teaspoons finely chopped fresh mint
(optional) Kosher salt and pepper to taste

DIRECTIONS

• Preheat the oven to 400 degrees.

• If the beets are very small, leave them whole. If
they are large, quarter them and lightly rub with
1 teaspoon olive oil. Place them in a roasting pan,
transfer to the oven and roast until they are soft
enough to be pierced with a fork, about 1 hour.

• Just prior to taking the beets out of the oven,
place the orange juice, vinegar, remaining olive
oil and mustard in a small pan and bring to a boil.
Gently peel the beets and pour this mixture over
them. Add salt and pepper to taste.

Mashed Sweet Potatoes

So naturally rich and wonderful, you'll think
you're eating dessert.

INGREDIENTS

• 4 sweet potatoes, peeled, if desired and diced 2
teaspoons unsalted butter

• 1 tablespoon honey or maple syrup (optional) Kosher salt, to taste

DIRECTIONS

• Place the potatoes in a large saucepan, cover with cold water and bring to a boil over high heat. Boil until the sweet potatoes are tender, about 20 minutes. Drain well, transfer to a bowl, add the butter and honey, if desired, and using a fork or a potato masher, mash until smooth. Add salt to taste. Serve immediately.

Basic Risotto

A classic Northern Italian dish, risotto is creamy and comforting. This version is much lower in fat than traditional recipes.

INGREDIENTS

• 1 teaspoon olive oil

• 1 medium Spanish onion, finely chopped 1 shallot, finely chopped

• 1 1/2 cups Arborio rice (Do not substitute any other kind) 4 1/2 - 5 cups non fat chicken or vegetable stock

• 6 ounces baby spinach

• Kosher salt and black pepper to taste Grated Parmesan Cheese, to taste

DIRECTIONS

• Place a large heavy bottomed saucepan over low heat and when it is hot, add the oil. Add the onion and cook until softened, 10-15 minutes.

• Add rice and sauté one minute. Add 1/2 cup stock to rice and simmer until all the stock has been absorbed, stirring constantly and slowly.

• Continue adding stock until all the stock has been absorbed, continuing to add it gradually and stirring all the while.

• Serve immediately, garnished with Parmesan cheese.

PASTA

Chunky Creamy Tomato Sauce

This creamy cream-less, vegetable laden tomato sauce is wonderful on pasta, quinoa, polenta and barley.

INGREDIENTS

- 1/4 cup water

- 2 garlic cloves, chopped

- 1 leek, very well washed or 1 small bunch scallions, trimmed and finely chopped 3 carrots, diced

- 2 tablespoons chopped fresh Italian flat leaf parsley leaves 1 28 ounce can diced tomatoes, including liquid

- 2 zucchini, diced

- 1 red bell pepper, seeded and diced 1/4 cup white wine or orange juice 1 teaspoon kosher salt

- 1/2 teaspoon black pepper 1/4 cup skim milk buttermilk 1/4 cup non fat Greek yogurt 1 tablespoon tomato paste

• 2 tablespoons chopped fresh basil leaves, plus additional for garnish 1 pound medium size shaped pasta, such as shells or rotini

DIRECTIONS

• Shaved or grated Parmesan cheese.

• Place the water, leek, scallions, garlic, carrots, parsley, tomatoes, zucchini and red pepper in a large non stick skillet over medium high heat and cook until the vegetables begin to soften, 10- 15 minutes.

• Add the wine or orange juice, salt and pepper and cook until all the vegetables are soft, about 20 minutes.

• Place the buttermilk, yogurt and tomato paste in a small bowl and stir to combine. Gradually add the buttermilk mixture to the skillet and cook for 2 - 3 minutes, stirring all the while. Stir in the basil.

• Bring a large pot of water to a boil and cook the pasta until al dente.

• Serve pasta in shallow bowls with sauce on top, garnished with Parmesan cheese.

Crave artichokes but don't want all the fuss? This pasta sauce includes artichoke hearts and bottoms for a rich, artichoke-y sauce. Be sure to rinse the artichokes well to get rid of any tinny flavor from the cans.

INGREDIENTS

- 3- 4 garlic cloves, thinly sliced

- 1 small onion, thinly sliced

- 1 16 ounce can artichoke hearts, drained, rinsed and chopped

- 1 16 ounce can artichoke bottoms, drained, rinsed and chopped 1 16 ounce can diced tomatoes, including juice

- 1 cup water

- Juice and zest of ½ lemon

- ¼ cup chopped fresh basil or parsley leaves

DIRECTIONS

• Place a large skillet over medium low heat and when it is hot, add the oil. Add the garlic and onion and cook until they are soft and golden, about 7 minutes. Raise the heat to medium high, add the artichoke hearts and cook, stirring occasionally, for five minutes. Add the tomatoes, and water and bring to a quick boil. Lower the heat to low, cover and cook 15 minutes. Add the lemon juice and zest and the basil. Serve immediately

Pasta with Broccoli Rabe and White Beans

The combination of the bitter broccoli rabe and the creamy white beans is heavenly. If you aren't a fan of broccoli rabe, feel free to substitute broccoli or cauliflower.

INGREDIENTS

• 2 teaspoons olive oil

• 4 garlic cloves, chopped or pressed

• 1 large bunch broccoli rabe, heavy stems removed and flowers coarsely chopped2 1/4 - 1/2 teaspoon crushed red pepper flakes (optional)

• 1 - 2 (16 ounce) cans white beans, drained and rinsed

• 1/2 pound medium sized, shaped pasta, such as penne, rigatoni or conchiglie

DIRECTIONS

• Place a large non stick skillet over medium heat and when it is hot, add the olive oil. Add the garlic and cook until just turning golden, about 2 minutes. Add the broccoli rabe, stir well and cook until the rabe begins to brighten, 3 - 5 minutes. Raise the heat to high, add red pepper flakes and white beans and cook until the beans are heated through, about 3 minutes.

• Bring a large pot of water to boil. Add pasta and cook until tender. Drain pasta, reserving 1/2 cup of pasta water. Add pasta water to broccoli rabe mixture and stir to combine. Add pasta and stir. Just prior to serving, add toasted pine nuts.

Pasta with Fresh Tomato Sauce

Dinner doesn't get any easier than this

• INGREDIENTS

- 1 pound dried pasta (any shape is fine) 1 teaspoon olive oil

- 2 garlic cloves, thinly sliced

- 2 28 ounce cans plum tomatoes, drained and coarsely chopped pinch

- white sugar

- 2 - 3 tablespoons water or wine 1 tablespoon dried basil

- 1 teaspoon dried oregano

- 1/4 cup fresh chopped basil leaves Shaved or grated Parmesan Cheese

DIRECTIONS

- Bring a large pot of water to boil. Add the pasta.

- Place a large non- stick skillet over medium heat and when it is hot, add the oil. Add the garlic and cook for 2 minutes. Add the tomatoes, sugar, water or wine, dried basil and oregano.

- Cook the tomato mixture until the pasta is tender, or about 15 minutes. Drain the pasta and place equal amounts on 4 plates and top with tomato sauce. Place fresh basil on top of each bowl. Serve immediately with fresh Parmesan cheese.

Pasta with Tomatoes and Arugula

Also known as rocket, roquette, rugula and rucola, arugula, aromatic and slightly bitter is a nice contrast to the tomatoes.

INGREDIENTS

- 1 teaspoon olive oil

- ¼ cup chopped Prosciutto (optional) 1

- small red onion, chopped

- 2 garlic cloves, minced

- 1 28 ounce can diced tomatoes, including the liquid

- 2 cups dry pasta

- 2 cups arugula, washed

- Grated Asiago or Parmesan cheese, for serving

DIRECTIONS

• Place a large pot of water over high heat and bring to a boil. Add the pasta and cook according to the package instructions or until al dente, about 12 minutes. Drain, reserving

• ½ cup pasta water.

• Place a large skillet over medium heat and add the oil. Add the onion and garlic and cook until soft, about 5 minutes. Add the tomatoes and cook 15 minutes. Add ½ cup pasta water. Add the pasta and cook until hot, about 1- 2 minutes.

• Place the arugula in the bottom of a large shallow bowl, top with the pasta mixture and toss gently. Serve immediately.

Pasta with Broccoli, Cauliflower and Toasted Pine Nuts

A wonderful and traditional classic Italian pasta dish for those who love vegetables in the cabbage family. Roasted Brussels sprouts could be exchanged for either the broccoli or cauliflower, walnuts for the pine nuts and dried cranberries for the raisins.

INGREDIENTS

• 2 teaspoons canola or olive oil

• 1 small Spanish onion, coarsely chopped 2 - 3 garlic cloves, finely chopped

• 1/2 head cauliflower, core removed, florets chopped

• 1/2 head broccoli, stem discarded or saved for another use, florets chopped 1 cup non fat chicken broth

• 1 pound medium sized, shaped pasta, such as penne, rigatoni or conchiglie 1/4 cup pine nuts, lightly toasted

• 1/2 cup raisins or currants

• 1/2 cup grated Parmesan cheese

• 1/2 cup chopped fresh Italian flat leaf parsley leaves 2 tablespoons balsamic vinegar

DIRECTIONS

• Place a large skillet over medium heat and when it is hot, add the oil. Add the onion and garlic and cook until the onion is golden, about 10 minutes.

• Add the cauliflower and broccoli florets and cook 5 minutes. Add the chicken broth and cook until the florets are almost tender, about 5 minutes.

• While the sauce is cooking, place the pine-nuts, raisins, parmesan cheese, parsley and balsamic vinegar in a bowl, toss together and set aside.

• Bring a large pot of water to boil. Add the pasta and cook until tender. Drain immediately and transfer to a shallow serving bowl. Add the broccoli mixture and top pine-nut mixture. Serve immediately.

Pasta with Roasted Bell Pepper Sauce

Roasting the bell peppers makes this sauce surprisingly delicate! Try it atop fish or chicken or even as a sandwich spread.

INGREDIENTS

• 6 red, orange or yellow bell peppers 4 garlic cloves

• 2 tablespoons olive oil

• 1 pound dried pasta (any shape is fine)

• 1/2 cup chopped Italian flat leaf parsley or basil leaves Parmesan cheese (optional)

DIRECTIONS

• Preheat broiler or oven to 500 degrees.

• Place the peppers directly under the broiler, as close together as possible and broil until blackened on all sides. Place the peppers in a heavy plastic or paper bag and let sweat for about 10 minutes. Remove burned skin. Seed and stem peppers.

• Place roasted peppers, garlic and olive oil in a food processor fitted with a steel blade and process until pureed.

• Bring a large pot of water to a boil. Add pasta and cook until al dente. Drain pasta, reserving 1/2- 1 cup of pasta water. Add pasta water to peppers and puree. Place equal amounts of pasta in 4 bowls and top with Roasted Pepper sauce. Garnish with the parsley or basil and Parmesan, if desired.

Pasta fagioli can be served as a first course, or an entree with a simple green salad and some bread.

INGREDIENTS

• 1 Spanish onion, chopped 2 celery stalks, chopped

• 2 carrots, chopped

• 2 garlic cloves, finely chopped or pressed 3 cups chicken stock nonfat

• 1 (28 ounce) can diced tomatoes

• 1 teaspoon dried or 1 tablespoon chopped fresh rosemary

• 4 cups cooked white cannellini beans, drained and rinsed

• 2 cups medium sized shaped pasta, such as penne, rigatoni or conchiglie

DIRECTIONS

• Place a large skillet over medium low heat, add the onion, celery, carrots, garlic and ¼ cup chicken stock. Cook until the vegetables are tender, about 20 minutes.

• Add the tomatoes and remaining stock. If you are using dried rosemary, add it now. Raise the heat to medium high and bring to a low boil. Reduce heat to low and cook for one hour.

• Add the beans and cook until heated throughout, 5 - 10 minutes.

• Bring a large pot of water to boil. Cook the pasta until al dente and transfer to a mixing bowl. Add the bean mixture and toss well. If you are using fresh rosemary, add it just prior to serving. Serve from the pot or place in a large ceramic bowl.

Broccoli Pesto

Instead of using fresh basil leaves, this pesto is made from broccoli, for a more nutritious sauce. While it was created to use on pasta, it also makes a great addition to barley, quinoa, rice and omelets and can also be used as a dip.

INGREDIENTS

• 1 small head broccoli, stems removed and saved for another use 2 garlic cloves, thinly sliced

• 1/3 cup grated Parmesan cheese

• 1 cup coarsely chopped fresh basil leaves Fill a large bowl with cold water.

DIRECTIONS

• Bring a large pot of water to a boil. Add the broccoli and garlic and boil until tender, about 20 minutes. Drain and place in the bowl with cold water. Drain and transfer to food processor fitted with a steel blade. Process until totally smooth, adding Parmesan and basil at the end.

• Serve immediately over just cooked pasta.

POULTRY AND FISH

Salmon with Mustard and Maple Syrup

A little bit of spice and a little bit of maple make this easy and quick salmon dish a perfect match for any dark green vegetable.

INGREDIENTS

- 1– 1 ¼ pound salmon filets, whole or divided into serving pieces 2 tablespoons Dijon mustard

- 2 tablespoons real Maple syrup 1 lemon or lime, quartered

INGREDIENTS

- Preheat the broiler.

- Place the salmon on a baking sheet and brush with the mustard and Maple syrup.

- Transfer to the broiler and cook until the salmon is deeply colored, about 6 minutes. Serve immediately, garnished with the lemon.

Salmon with Balsamic, Orange and Rosemary

If fresh rosemary isn't available, don't even think of substituting dried rosemary. Instead try fresh basil or cilantro. Serve with steamed rice, quinoa or barley and a dark green vegetable.

INGREDIENTS

- ¼ cup orange juice

- ¼ cup balsamic vinegar

- 1 – 1 ¼ pounds salmon filet, whole or cut into serving pieces 1 teaspoon fresh rosemary leaves

- 1 tablespoon finely chopped chives

DIRECTIONS

- Place the orange juice and balsamic vinegar in a small pan and bring to a boil over high heat. Continue cooking until the liquid has halved, about 5 minutes. Set aside while you prepare the salmon.

- To cook the salmon: Place a large non-stick pan over medium high heat and when it is hot, add the salmon. Cook until it begins to color, 3- 4 minutes on each side. Add the orange juice mixture and rosemary and cook for 1 minute. Serve immediately, garnished with the chives.

Salmon Steaks with Herbs

These herby salmon steaks are a fantastic welcome for the spring grilling season. Try the herb paste on boneless chicken, too.

INGREDIENTS

For the herbs:

- 1 tablespoons fresh basil leaves

- 2 tablespoons fresh cilantro leaves

- ¼ cup Italian flat leaf parsley leaves

- 2 tablespoons water

- 1 garlic clove

- 1 teaspoon dried oregano

- For the salmon:

- 1 tablespoon olive oil

- 4 6-ounce salmon steaks, ¾- 1 inch thick 1 teaspoon kosher salt

- ½ teaspoon black pepper

DIRECTIONS

- To make the herb mixture: Place all the ingredients in a food processor fitted with a steel blade and process until fully chopped and as smooth as you can get it.

- To cook the salmon: Place a large skillet over high heat and when it is hot, add oil. Add the salmon and cook until deeply browned, about 5 minutes on each side. Top with the herb mixture and serve immediately.

Turkey Chili

This makes a large batch, enough for a party or enough to serve for dinner and then have leftovers for the freezer: freeze in individual containers for a quick lunch or dinner. The alcohol will cook off the beer but if you don't want to include, simply omit it. If the chili gets too thick, simply add a little bit of water.

Good accompaniments include chopped fresh basil or cilantro, chopped scallions, non- fat plain yogurt, chopped tomatoes, fresh lime quarters... the list is almost endless!

INGREDIENTS

• 2 Spanish onions, finely chopped (about 4 cups) 1 red bell pepper, cut into 1/2-inch cubes

• 6 garlic cloves, minced 1/4 cup chili powder

• 1 tablespoon ground cumin

• 1 teaspoon crushed red pepper flakes 1 teaspoon dried Greek oregano

- 1/2 teaspoon cayenne 1 bottle beer or ale

- 2 pounds ground turkey

- 2 cans (16 ounces each) black turtle beans, drained and rinsed 1

- can (28 ounces) diced tomatoes, with juice 1 can (28 ounces) can tomato puree

DIRECTIONS

- Place a large non-stick stockpot over medium heat, add the onion, garlic, peppers, chili powder, cumin, red pepper flakes, oregano, cayenne and ¼ cup beer and cook, stirring occasionally, until all have softened but not browned, 15- 20 minutes. Add the ground turkey and cook, breaking it up with a wooden spoon, until it loses its rawness, about 5 minutes. Add the remaining beer, beans, tomatoes and tomato puree and bring to a gentle boil. Lower the heat to low and cook until the chili starts to come together, about 2 hours. Set aside to cool for 20 minutes. Transfer to a container, cover and refrigerate overnight. Reheat gently over low to medium heat.

The classic combination of mustard, apple and pork makes this dish comfort food. For even more apple, serve this with fresh applesauce.

INGREDIENTS

• boneless pork chops, about 1 ½ pounds total 1 teaspoon kosher salt

• ½ teaspoon black pepper 1 teaspoon olive oil

• 3 tablespoons Dijon mustard 2/3 cup apple cider

DIRECTIONS

• Place a non-stick skillet over medium high heat and when it is hot, add the oil. Sprinkle the pork chops with the salt and pepper and place in the pan. Cook until lightly browned, 4- 7 minutes on each side, depending on the thickness. Transfer the chops to a platter and add the mustard and apple cider to the pan. Bring to a boil and pour over the chops. Serve immediately.

Savory and sweet, serve these pork chops with roasted squash or sweet potatoes and steamed rice.

INGREDIENTS

- 1 teaspoon kosher salt

- ½ teaspoon black pepper

- ½ teaspoon coarsely ground dried fennel 1 teaspoon fresh rosemary leaves

- 2 teaspoons olive oil

- 4 boneless pork chops, about 1 1/2 pounds total 2 garlic cloves, minced

- 1/2- 2/3 cup fresh orange juice

- 1 tablespoon apricot or peach jam

DIRECTIONS

- Place the salt, pepper, fennel and rosemary on a plate and mix to combine. Dredge the pork chops in the mixture, pressing the mixture into them.

• Place a large non-stick skillet over medium high heat and when it is hot, add 1 teaspoon oil. Add the pork chops and cook until well browned, about 4- 5 minutes on each side. Transfer the chops to a plate and cover with aluminum foil. Lower the heat to low, add the remaining 1 teaspoon oil and when it is hot, add the garlic. When the garlic is just golden, add the juice and jam. Bring to a boil and cook, stirring, for 2 minutes. Return the chops to the pan and cook for 1 minute. Serve immediately.

TUNA AU POIVRE

Peppery, herby and lemony.

INGREDIENTS

• 1 tablespoon finely grated lemon zest

• 3 - 4 teaspoons coarsely ground black pepper 2 garlic cloves, finely minced

• 2 teaspoons dried oregano 1 teaspoon kosher salt

• 4 6 ounce tuna

• steaks 2 teaspoons olive oil 1 lemon, quartered

DIRECTIONS

• Place the lemon zest, black pepper, garlic, oregano and salt on a large plate and mix to combine. Dredge both sides of the tuna in the mixture.

• Place a large cast iron skillet over medium high heat and when it is hot, add the oil. Add the tuna and cook until browned, about 5 minutes on each side.

• Serve immediately, garnished with the lemon quarters.

Fish Stew

Serve this heady stew with steamed rice or French bread.

INGREDIENTS

• 2 teaspoons olive oil

• 3 leeks, well washed, white and light green parts only, or 1 Spanish onion, chopped 2 celery stalks, diced

• 2 carrots, diced peeled

• 1 fennel bulb, tough outer layers removed, trimmed and diced 4 garlic cloves, finely chopped or pressed

• 1/4 teaspoon crushed red pepper 2 teaspoons dried thyme

• 1 bay leaf

• 1/4 teaspoon cayenne pepper

• 1/8 teaspoon crushed saffron threads

• 1 28 ounce can whole tomatoes, chopped, including liquid 6 cups light fish broth or non-fat chicken broth

• 1 cup dry white wine

• Strips of zest from one orange 1 pound cod, cubed

• 1 pound halibut, cubed

DIRECTIONS

• Place a large skillet over low heat and when it is hot, add the olive oil. Add the onion, celery, carrots and fennel and cook until the onion is golden, about 10 minutes.

• Add garlic, herbs and spices and cook for 5 minutes. Add tomatoes, fish broth, wine and orange zest and cook for 20- 25 minutes.

• Raise the heat to high and bring the mixture to a boil. Reduce the heat to low, add the cod and halibut and cook until the fish is starting to fall part, 10- 15 minutes.

• Transfer 2 cups of the soup to a blender and process until smooth. Return to the soup. Serve immediately or cover and refrigerate up to 2 days. Serve with lemon wedges and French bread toasts or croutons.

Grilled Salmon with Fruit and Sesame Vinaigrette

There are a ton of ingredients in this dish but after you make it once, you'll see it's well worth it.

INGREDIENTS

• 4 6-ounce salmon

• steaks 1 teaspoon kosher salt

• 1 teaspoon black pepper 1 teaspoon olive oil

- 1 garlic clove, crushed

- 1 teaspoon finely chopped fresh ginger root peeled

- ½ cup chopped red onion 2 tablespoons sesame seeds 1/4 cup lemon or lime juice

- ¼ cup orange, apple or pineapple juice

- ¼ teaspoon white sugar

- 1 tablespoon balsamic vinegar

- 1 tablespoon finely chopped fresh basil or cilantro leaves 2 scallion greens, finely chopped

- ¼- ½ teaspoon kosher salt

DIRECTIONS

- Prepare the grill or preheat the broiler.

- Sprinkle the salmon with the salt and pepper. When the grill is hot, place the steaks on the grill and cook 5- 6 minutes on each side. Alternatively, place under the broiler.

- In the meantime, place a large skillet over medium heat and when it is hot, add the oil. Add the garlic, ginger root, onion and sesame seeds and cook until the vegetables are soft and the seeds are lightly browned, about 5 minutes. Off heat, add the juices, sugar, vinegar, basil or cilantro, scallion greens, salt and pepper.

• When the steaks are ready, top with the vinaigrette. Serve immediately.

Roasted Chicken

If you know how to cook only one thing, this is it. Feel free to add hard vegetables like potatoes, onions, shallots, carrots, sweet potatoes, turnips, beets and butternut squash to the pan while you roast the chicken. You can also stuff the cavities with fresh rosemary, thyme or parsley leaves and/or lemon, apple or onions, or a combination.

INGREDIENTS

• 1 whole roaster chicken, about 6 - 7 pounds 1 - 1 1/2 teaspoons kosher salt

• 1/4 teaspoon black pepper

DIRECTIONS

• Preheat oven to 450 degrees. Remove and discard giblets and neck from chicken cavity.

Rinse chicken in several changes of cold water and pat dry.

• Rub skin and flesh with kosher salt and black pepper. Place on roasting rack in pan. Transfer to oven and roast the juices run clear from the breast and the leg moves easily and the internal temperature is about 160 degrees, about 70 minutes (10 minutes per pound).

• Do not baste. Cut the chicken into serving pieces and remove the skin.

Turkey Meatloaf

This lighter meatloaf is great for dinner but equally delicious leftover in a sandwich.

INGREDIENTS

• 1 teaspoon olive oil

• 1 small Spanish onion, chopped

• 2- 3 garlic cloves, finely chopped or pressed 1 teaspoon dried Greek oregano

• 2 - 3 tablespoons Dijon mustard 1/2 teaspoon black pepper

- 1/4 - 1/2 teaspoon salt

- 3/4 cup tomato ketchup or barbecue sauce

- 1/2 cup chopped fresh Italian flat leaf parsley leaves 2 slices good quality white bread

- 1/2 cup beef or chicken stock none fat

- 1 large egg, lightly beaten

- 2 pounds lean ground chicken or turkey

DIRECTIONS

- Preheat the oven to 350 degrees. Lightly grease an 8 x 4 inch loaf pan.

- Place a medium size skillet over low heat and when it is hot, add the oil. Add the onion, garlic and oregano and cook until the onion is golden, about 10 minutes.

- Transfer to a large mixing bowl and set aside to cool.

- In the meantime, soak the bread in the stock until it is moist, about 2 minutes. Drain off as much liquid as possible. Add the bread to the cooled onion mixture.

• Add the eggs and ground meat and mix, by hand , until everything is thoroughly incorporated. Place the mixture in the prepared loaf pan, transfer to the oven and cook for about 1 hour and 15 minutes.

Vietnamese Style Chicken

Steamed green beans and brown rice complete this to make a great weekday dinner.

INGREDIENTS

• 2 tablespoons plus 1/3 cup water

• ¼ cup Asian fish sauce

• 2 large shallots or 1 small onion, finely chopped 2 garlic cloves, minced

• Pinch black pepper

• Pinch crushed red pepper flakes

• ¼ cup sugar

• 1 ½ pounds boneless skinless chicken breasts (2 large), each breast half cut in half

• ¼ cup chopped fresh basil or cilantro leaves

DIRECTIONS

• Place the 2 tablespoons water and Asian fish sauce in a small bowl and set aside. Place the shallots, garlic, black and red peppers in another small bowl and set aside.

• Place the remaining 1/3 cup water and the sugar in a large skillet and cook over medium heat until the sugar has caramelized into a deep brown, about 6 minutes.

• Remove the pan from the heat, and .very carefully (to avoid splattering) add the fish sauce mixture to the pan. Return to the heat and cook until the mixture boils. 1-2 minutes. Add the shallot mixture and cook until the shallots have softened, about 3 minutes. Add the chicken, in a single layer, and cook, stirring occasionally, until cooked throughout, about 4 minutes per side. Serve immediately, sprinkled with the basil.

Pan Grilled Chicken with Lemon and Basil

Serve with steamed brown or white rice and a chopped tomato salad.

INGREDIENTS

* 1 ½ pounds boneless, skinless chicken breasts, pounded thin and sliced lengthwise to get 4 cutlets

* ¼ cup fresh lemon juice

* ¼ cup chopped fresh basil leaves 1 teaspoon dried oregano

* ½ teaspoon black pepper

* ½ teaspoon kosher salt

DIRECTIONS

* Place the chicken, lemon juice, basil and oregano in a non-reactive glass or ceramic bowl and mix to combine. Cover and refrigerate at least 2 but no more than 4 hours.

* Drain the chicken and discard the marinade. Sprinkle with the salt and pepper.

* Place a large cast iron skillet over medium high heat and when it is almost smoking hot, add the chicken, waiting for the pan to reheat between additions. Cook until golden brown, just firm to the touch and cooked throughout, about 4 minutes per side, depending on the thickness of the chicken.

Grilled Pineapple

A superb dessert to make when you already have the grill going, this low-calorie, low- fat treat is easy and impressive.

INGREDIENTS

• 1 tablespoon unsalted butter 2 teaspoons brown sugar Juice of ½ lime

• 1 fresh pineapple, cored and cut into eighths, lengthwise

DIRECTIONS

• Place the butter, brown sugar and lime juice in a small bowl and mix well. Prepare a grill or preheat the broiler.

• Brush butter mixture on the pineapple, place on the grill or under the broiler and cook, turning once, until lightly browned on both sides, about 4 minutes. Drizzle with the remaining butter mixture.

You don't need an ice cream machine to make this incredibly easy and quick dessert. You do, however, need to keep an arsenal of frozen fruit in the freezer. You can substitute the peaches with any kind of berry, mangoes, papayas or simply add more bananas, or jazz it up with ground cinnamon or nutmeg. For those who want something a little sweeter, swirl in any flavor of unsweetened fruit spread.

INGREDIENTS

• 2 over - ripe bananas, thinly sliced and frozen

• 2 cups chopped fresh peaches, peeled, if desired and frozen

• ½ teaspoon vanilla extract

• 1/3 cup plain low-fat yogurt

DIRECTIONS

• Place the frozen bananas and peaches in the bowl of a food processor fitted with a steel blade. Process until smooth. Gradually add the vanilla and yogurt and process until completely incorporated. Serve immediately.

Tart, sweet, warm and comforting, these apples can be served hot, cold or at room temperature. Feel free to use any variety of apple you like.

INGREDIENTS

- 1 tablespoon maple syrup

- 1/2 teaspoon ground cinnamon

- 1/4 cup raisins or currants 1/3 cup orange juice

- 2 strips lemon zest, grated or chopped (optional)

- 4 Granny Smith apples, cored and top third cut off and discarded

DIRECTIONS

- Preheat the oven to 375 degrees.

- Place the maple syrup, cinnamon, raisins and, if desired, the lemon peel, in a small bowl and mix well. Place apples in a small baking dish, so that they touch each other .Divide the maple syrup mixture into four parts and stuff inside apples. Pour the orange juice around them.

• Transfer to the oven and bake until the apples
are soft, about one hour.

Fragrant and sweet, this quick dessert will scent
your home and impress your family and friends.

INGREDIENTS

• 2 firm pears, peeled, quartered and cored 2
tablespoons maple syrup

• 2 teaspoons lemon juice

• ½ teaspoon vanilla extract Pinch ground
cinnamon Pinch kosher salt

DIRECTIONS

• Preheat the oven to 400 degrees. Line a baking
sheet with parchment paper or a silpat.

• Place everything in a bowl and toss well. Place
the pears on the baking sheet and drizzle with
the remaining liquid. Transfer to the oven and
roast until deep brown and tender, 30 minutes.

Broiled Grapefruit with Mint and Honey

A very old fashioned dessert that is making a comeback, Broiled Grapefruit is a nice way to enjoy fruit.

INGREDIENTS

• 2 large grapefruits, halved, large seeds removed 1 tablespoon honey or maple syrup

• Mint leaves, for garnish

DIRECTIONS

• Place the grapefruits, cut side up, on a large baking sheet. Drizzle with the honey and transfer to the broiler. Broil until the top is browned and bubbling, about 5 minutes. Set aside for 3- 4 minutes and serve, garnished with mint leaves.

Rhubarb Strawberry Compote

This classic combination heralds spring! If you are lucky enough to have rhubarb growing in your backyard, be sure to freeze enough to make this compote year-round.

INGREDIENTS

- 4 cups washed, trimmed and chopped rhubarb stalks, remove and discard the leaves 3 cups chopped strawberries

- 1 teaspoon cornstarch

- 1 tablespoon brown sugar 1 teaspoon fresh lemon zest

DIRECTIONS

- Place the rhubarb, berries and cornstarch in a medium saucepan and cook over medium heat until it reaches a low boil, about 7 minutes. Lower the heat to low and cook until the rhubarb is soft and the mixture has thickened, about 30 minutes. Off heat, add the sugar and lemon zest.

- Serve warm or at room temperature

Apple Banana sauce

Created as a use for over-ripe bananas, Apple Banana sauce has become a beloved dessert, snack, even breakfast parfaited with Greek yogurt.

INGREDIENTS

• 3 tart apples, cored, peeled and sliced 3 over-ripe bananas

• 1 teaspoon ground cinnamon

DIRECTIONS

• Place the apples in the bowl of a food processor fitted with a steel blade and process until they are well chopped. Scrape down the sides of the bowl and add the banana and cinnamon. Process until smooth. Transfer to a bowl, cover and refrigerate at least one and up to four hours.